Frankincense Essential Oil

The Ultimate Guide to Frankincense Essential Oil with 25 Recipes

Table of Contents

Introduction

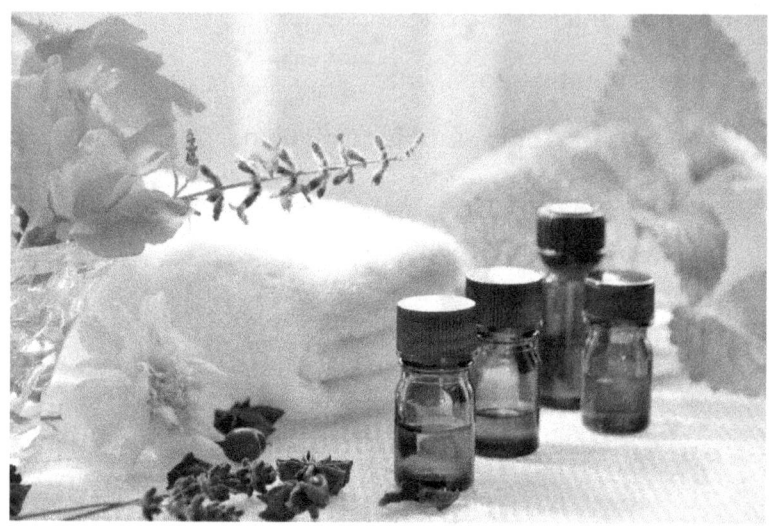

Essential oils can be extracted from a wide variety of plants and plant products. These oils contain the volatile aroma compounds, or the "essence" of the plant from which they are derived. Not only do essential oils capture the fragrance of the plant, but they also contain the compounds that are responsible for any medicinal benefits the plant has to offer. Essential oils have been used in a variety of different cultures for thousands of years as part of natural remedies, perfumes, cosmetics and more.

Though there are hundreds of different essential oils out there, one of the oldest and most frequently used oil is frankincense essential oil. This oil offers a great many benefits for skin, hair, healing, and even mental health – it all depends how you use it. If you are curious to learn more about this wonderful oil, this book is the perfect place to start. Within the pages of this book you will receive an introduction to frankincense essential oil including what it is, where it comes from, and what kind of benefits it has to offer. You will also receive a collection of recipes for using frankincense essential oil.

What is Frankincense Essential Oil?

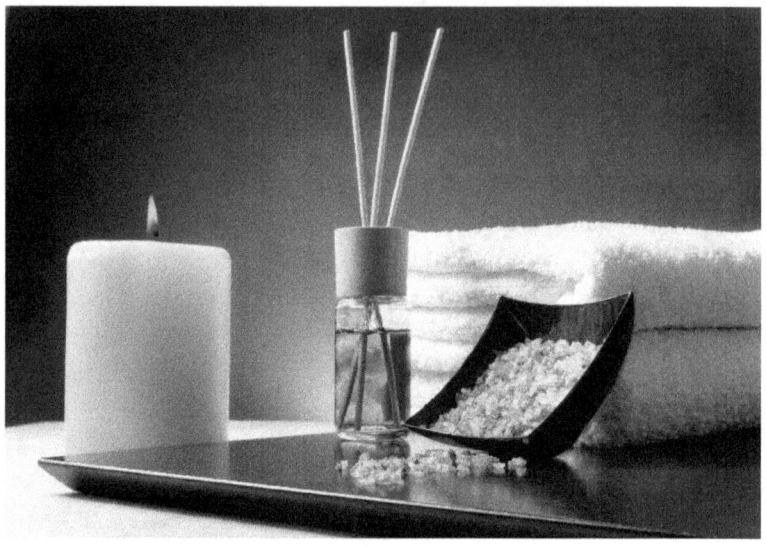

Frankincense is also known as olibanum, and it is not a type of plant – it is an aromatic resin that comes from a plant. The resin that forms frankincense comes from a certain genus of trees called Boswellia. There are four main species – the resin derived from each type of tree comes in different grades according to when the resin was harvested. Frankincense essential oil is produced through steam distillation of the dry resin, and it is frequently used in aromatherapy and perfumery. This essential oil has an uplifting, earthy aroma that is said to elevate spiritual experiences.

Uses and Benefits for Frankincense Essential Oil

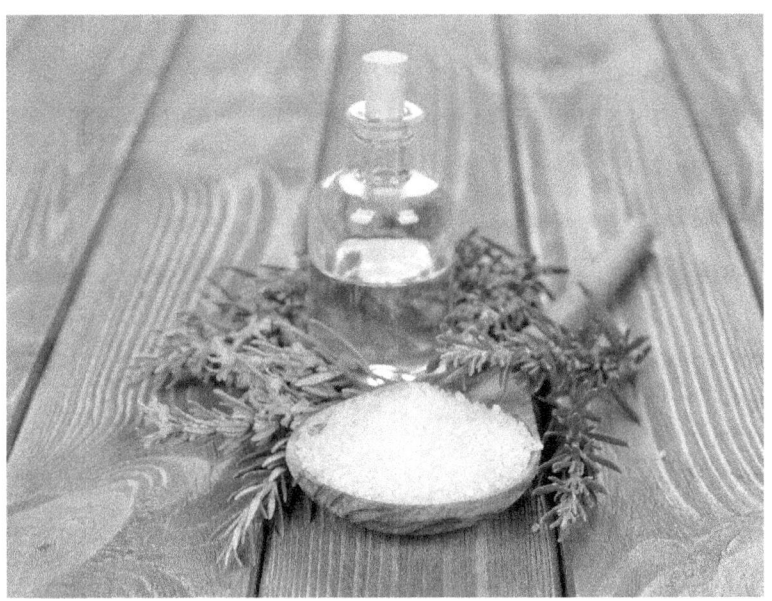

Frankincense essential oil has been used for thousands of years in a variety of different cultures. In the Middle East, this essential oil is commonly used during religious ceremonies, particularly as an anointing oil. In ancient Egyptian and Anglo-Saxon cultures, the oil has been a popular ingredient in cosmetics and perfumery. This essential oil is particularly well-known for its calming and soothing properties and it is thought to enhance spiritual connections. Frankincense essential oil may also help with stress and despair. Additionally, frankincense essential oil may provide certain skin benefits, promoting cellular regeneration and acting as a treatment for dry skin. When used properly, frankincense essential oil may help reverse the signs of aging and it can even speed healing, reducing the appearance of stretch marks and scars. This oil can also be used to strengthen the gums and roots of the hair – it may also help stop wounds from bleeding.

Frankincense Essential Oil Recipes

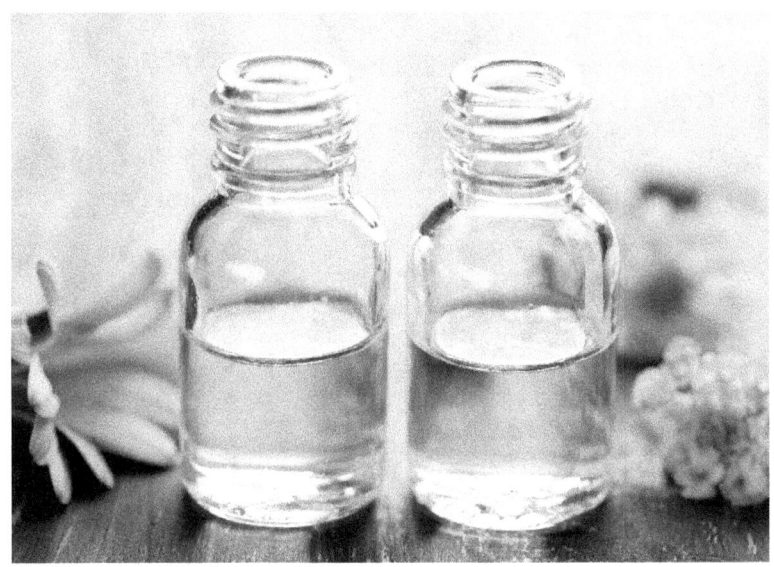

Recipes Included in this Book:

Simply Spiced Bath Salts

Healing Lip Balm

Cleansing Facial Cream

Depression-Lifting
Diffuser Blend

Anti-Inflammatory
Massage Oil

Soothing Frankincense
Bath Oil

Antiseptic Room Spray

Pain-Relieving Salve for
Joints and Muscles

Spiced Orange Bath Salts

Meditation-Boosting
Inhalation

Anti-Aging Facial
Cleanser

Restful Massage Oil for Insomnia

Concentration-Boosting Room Spray

Lovely Lavender Bath Salts

Feeling Free Diffuser Blend

Frankincense Healing Salve for Burns and Cuts

Restful Relaxation Bath Oil

Mood-Balancing Massage Oil

Spiritual Awakening Bath Salts

Nerve-Calming Inhalation

Sleep-Promoting Room Spray

Frankincense Toothpaste for Oral Pain

Moisturizing Floral Facial Cream

Pain-Relieving Bath Oil Blend

Immune-Boosting Diffuser Blend

Simply Spiced Bath Salts

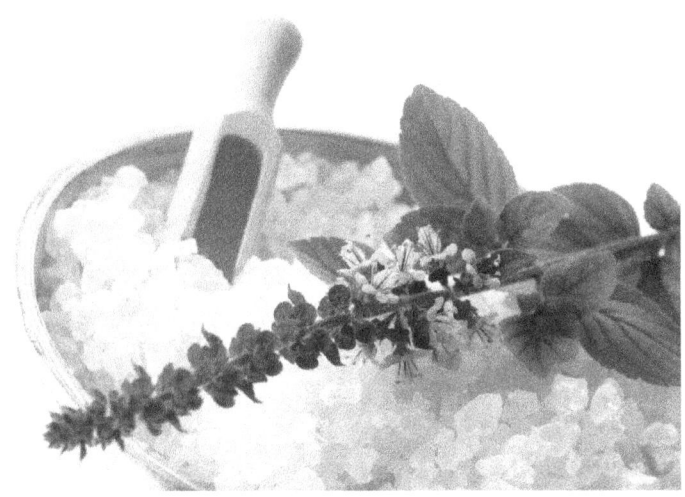

Ingredients:

- 2 cups Epsom salts
- 1 cup coarse Himalayan pink salt
- ½ cup baking soda
- 5 drops frankincense essential oil
- 3 drops patchouli essential oil
- 1 drop vetiver essential oil

Instructions:

1. Combine the Epsom salts, Himalayan salt and baking soda in a large bowl.
2. Stir until well combined then add the essential oils.
3. Use a metal spoon to stir the ingredients together then store in a dark glass jar.

4. Cover the jar with the lid and let the oils blend for at least 24 hours
5. To use the bath salts, draw a hot bath and stir in 1 cup of bath salt until thoroughly dissolved.
6. Soak for at least 30 minutes then towel dry.

Healing Lip Balm

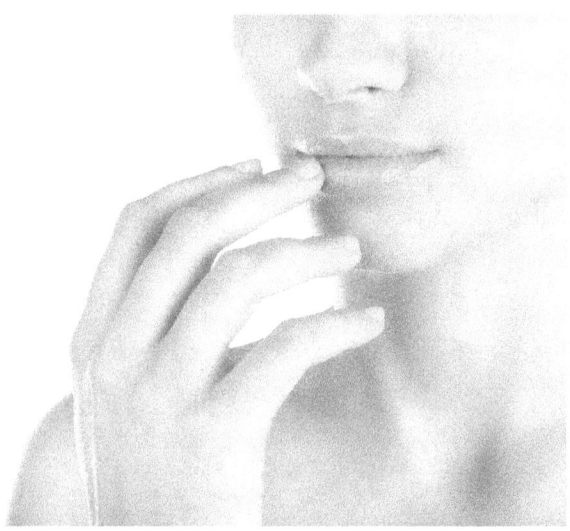

Ingredients:

- 1 tablespoon shea butter
- 1 tablespoon cold-pressed coconut oil
- ½ tablespoon beeswax granules
- 4 drops frankincense essential oil
- 3 drops grapefruit essential oil
- 3 drops rosemary essential oil

Instructions:

1. Combine the shea butter, coconut oil and beeswax in a double boiler over low heat.
2. Heat until the ingredients are melted then remove from heat.
3. Stir in the essential oils until thoroughly combined.

4. Fill empty lip chap containers with the mixture or pour it into small glass jars.
5. Let the mixture solidify at room temperature then store in a cool, dry place.

Cleansing Facial Cream

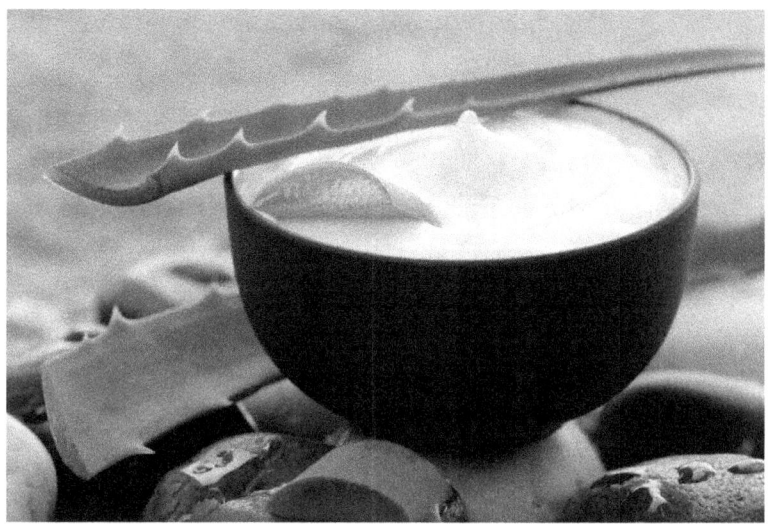

Ingredients:

- 6 tablespoons sweet almond oil
- 2 tablespoons emulsifying wax
- 2 tablespoons vegetable glycerin
- ½ teaspoon stearic acid
- 1 teaspoon vitamin E oil
- 8 tablespoons geranium hydrosol
- 4 tablespoons rose hydrosol, or rose water
- 2 tablespoons aloe vera gel
- 8 to 12 drops grapefruit seed extract
- 8 drops frankincense essential oil
- 8 drops patchouli essential oil
- 2 drops geranium essential oil

Instructions:

1. Combine the sweet almond oil, emulsifying wax, vegetable glycerin and stearic acid in a double boiler over low heat.
2. Warm the mixture until the wax melts then remove from heat.
3. Stir in the vitamin E oil then set aside to cool.
4. In a microwave-safe bowl, combine the hydrosols with the aloe vera gel.
5. Warm the mixture until it is lukewarm then stir it into the oil mixture.
6. Add the essential oils and grapefruit seed extract, stirring well.
7. Pour the mixture into an 8-ounce dark glass bottle and cool to room temperature.
8. Put the lid on the jar and store in a cool, dark area – shake before using.

Depression-Lifting Diffuser Blend

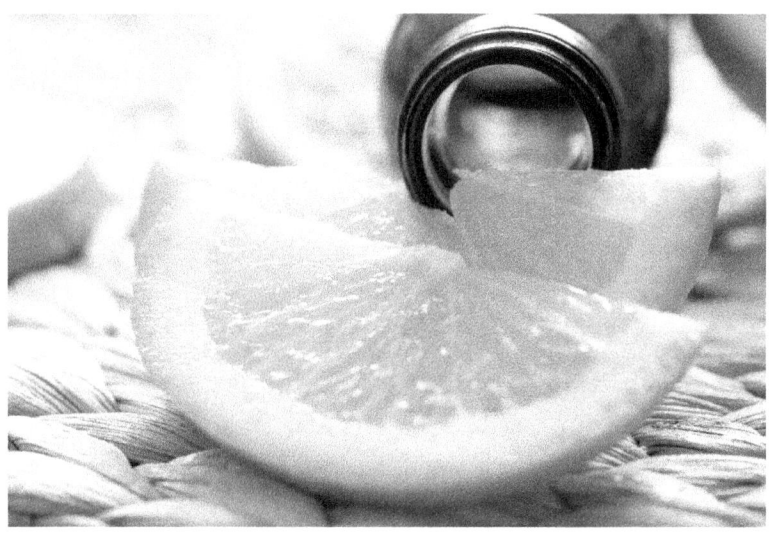

Ingredients:

- ¼ cup sweet almond oil
- 1 tablespoon high-proof vodka
- ½ teaspoon frankincense essential oil
- ¼ teaspoon bergamot essential oil
- ¼ teaspoon clary sage essential oil

Instructions:

1. Combine the sweet almond oil, vodka, and essential oils in a glass bottle.
2. Place the cap on the bottle and swirl gently to combine the ingredients.
3. Remove the cap and place several diffuser reeds in the bottle.

4. Let the reeds soak until saturated then turn them over to put the dry ends in the bottle.

Anti-Inflammatory Massage Oil

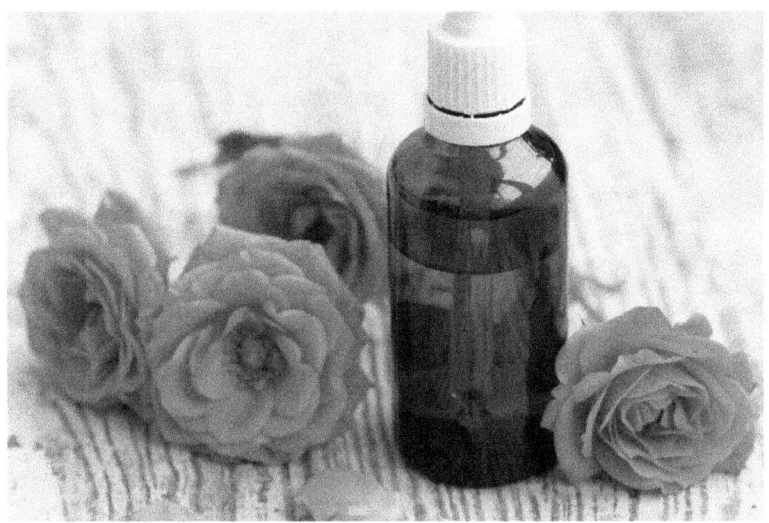

Ingredients:

- ¼ cup jojoba oil
- 5 drops frankincense essential oil
- 2 drops rose essential oil
- 2 drops eucalyptus essential oil

Instructions:

1. Combine the ingredients in a dark glass bottle.
2. Swirl gently to combine the oils then store with the lid on.
3. Let the oils blend for 24 hours then test for fragrance.
4. Apply the massage oil to bare skin and massage it in by hand.

Soothing Frankincense Bath Oil

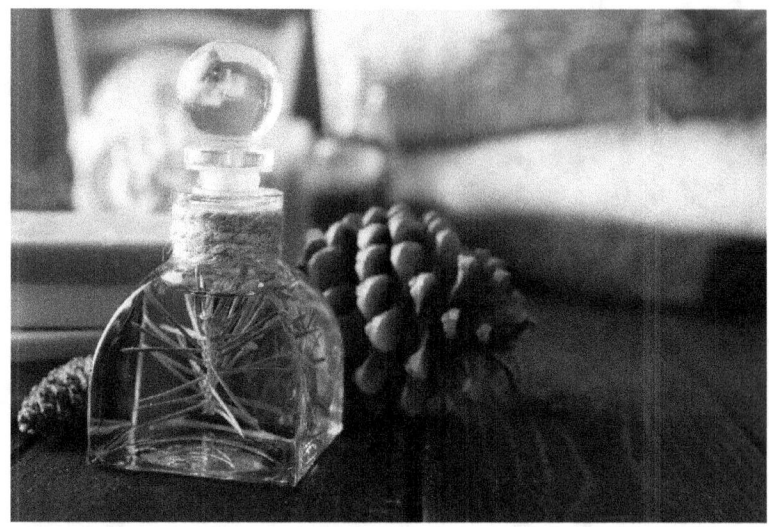

Ingredients:

- 8 drops lavender essential oil
- 6 drops frankincense essential oil
- 4 drops sweet marjoram essential oil
- 2 drops cedarwood essential oil
- ½ cup jojoba oil

Instructions:

1. Combine all of the essential oils in a small dark glass bottle.
2. Swirl the oils gently to combine then add the jojoba oil and swirl again.
3. To use the oils, run a hot bath then add up to 1 tablespoon of the bath oil.

4. Stir the water gently by hand to disperse the oils.
5. Soak for at least 30 minutes then towel dry.

Antiseptic Room Spray

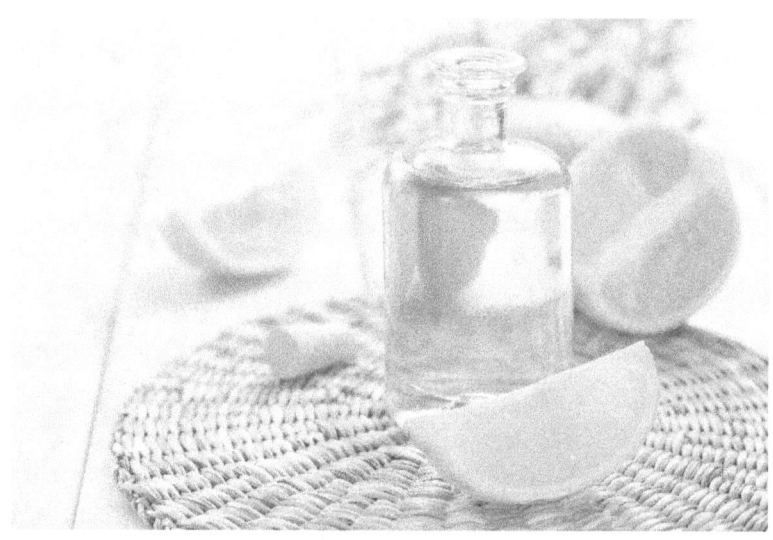

Ingredients:

- 2 tablespoons high-proof vodka
- 10 drops bergamot essential oil
- 10 drops tea tree essential oil
- 5 drops frankincense essential oil
- 5 drops lemon essential oil

Instructions:

1. Combine the vodka and essential oils in a small spray bottle.
2. Add the water then shake well to combine.
3. Spritz the spray into the air as needed.

Pain-Relieving Salve for Joints and Muscles

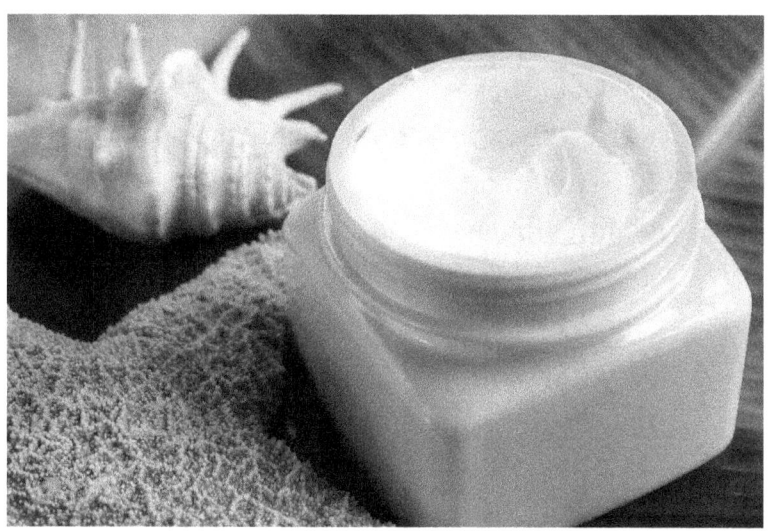

Ingredients:

- 1 cup organic olive oil
- 1 ounce dried oregano, ginger, and comfrey
- ½ ounce beeswax granules
- 1 vitamin E oil capsule
- ¼ teaspoon frankincense essential oil
- 6 drops basil essential oil
- 6 drops marjoram essential oil
- 6 drops rosemary essential oil

Instructions:

1. Combine the olive oil and herbs in a double boiler over low heat.
2. Warm the mixture to simmering and let simmer for 3 hours.
3. Strain the oil through a sieve back into the top of the double boiler.
4. Add the beeswax and warm until the wax is melted then stir smooth.
5. Remove from heat and stir in the vitamin E oil and essential oils.
6. Pour in the melted mixture into a small glass jar.
7. Let the jar set at room temperature until it solidifies.
8. Use the salve as needed for burns, cuts, and other minor injuries.

Spiced Orange Bath Salts

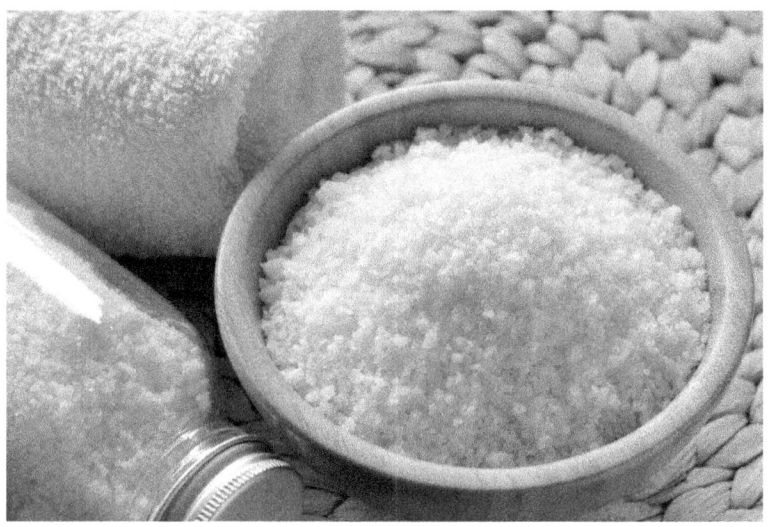

Ingredients:

- 2 cups Epsom salts
- 1 cup coarse sea salt
- ½ cup baking soda
- 4 drops frankincense essential oil
- 4 drops bergamot essential oil
- 1 drop ginger essential oil

Instructions:

1. Combine the Epsom salts, sea salt and baking soda in a large bowl.
2. Stir until well combined then add the essential oils.
3. Use a metal spoon to stir the ingredients together then store in a dark glass jar.

4. Cover the jar with the lid and let the oils blend for at least 24 hours
5. To use the bath salts, draw a hot bath and stir in 1 cup of bath salt until thoroughly dissolved.
6. Soak for at least 30 minutes then towel dry.

Meditation-Boosting Inhalation

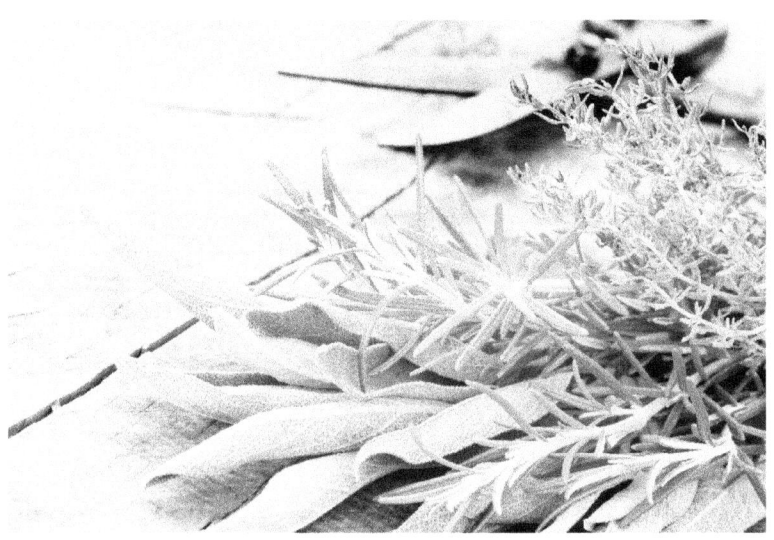

Ingredients:

- 2 to 3 drops frankincense essential oil
- 2 to 3 drops sage essential oil

Instructions:

1. Add the essential oil drops to a clean cloth or tissue.
2. Place the cloth under your nose and inhale deeply during meditation.

Anti-Aging Facial Cleanser

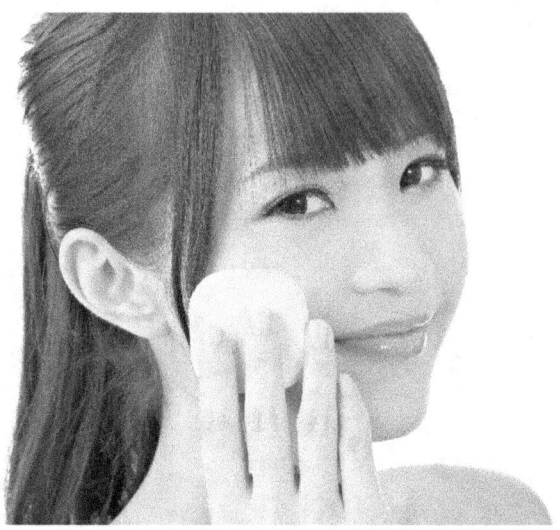

Ingredients:

- 6 tablespoons jojoba oil
- 2 tablespoons emulsifying wax
- 3 tablespoons vegetable glycerin
- ½ teaspoon stearic acid
- 1 teaspoon vitamin E oil
- 6 tablespoons geranium hydrosol
- 6 tablespoons rose hydrosol, or rose water
- 2 tablespoons aloe vera gel
- 9 drops grapefruit seed extract
- 8 drops geranium essential oil
- 5 drops frankincense essential oil
- 2 drops sandalwood essential oil

- 1 drop rose essential oil

Instructions:

1. Combine the jojoba oil, emulsifying wax, vegetable glycerin and stearic acid in a double boiler over low heat.
2. Warm the mixture until the wax melts then remove from heat.
3. Stir in the vitamin E oil then set aside to cool.
4. In a microwave-safe bowl, combine the hydrosols with the aloe vera gel.
5. Warm the mixture until it is lukewarm then stir it into the oil mixture.
6. Add the essential oils and grapefruit seed extract, stirring well.
7. Pour the mixture into an 8-ounce dark glass bottle and cool to room temperature.
8. Put the lid on the jar and store in a cool, dark area – shake before using.

Restful Massage Oil for Insomnia

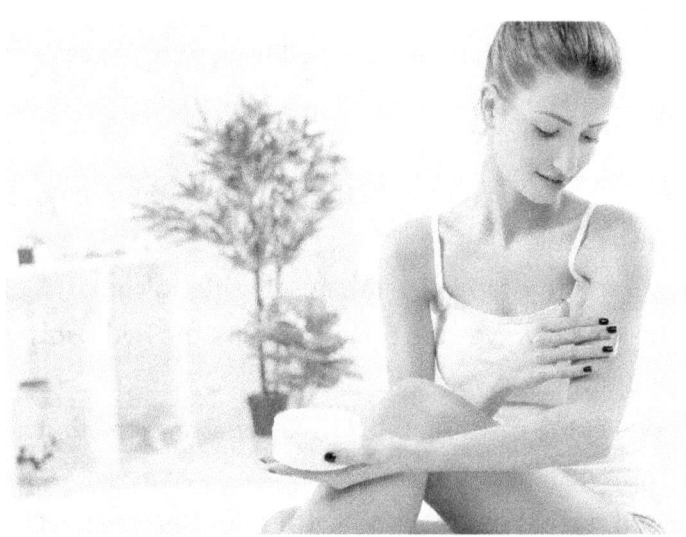

Ingredients:

- ¼ cup jojoba oil
- 4 drops frankincense essential oil
- 2 drops sandalwood essential oil
- 2 drops clary sage essential oil

Instructions:

1. Combine the ingredients in a dark glass bottle.
2. Swirl gently to combine the oils then store with the lid on.
3. Let the oils blend for 24 hours then test for fragrance.
4. Apply the massage oil to bare skin and massage it in by hand.

Concentration-Boosting Room Spray

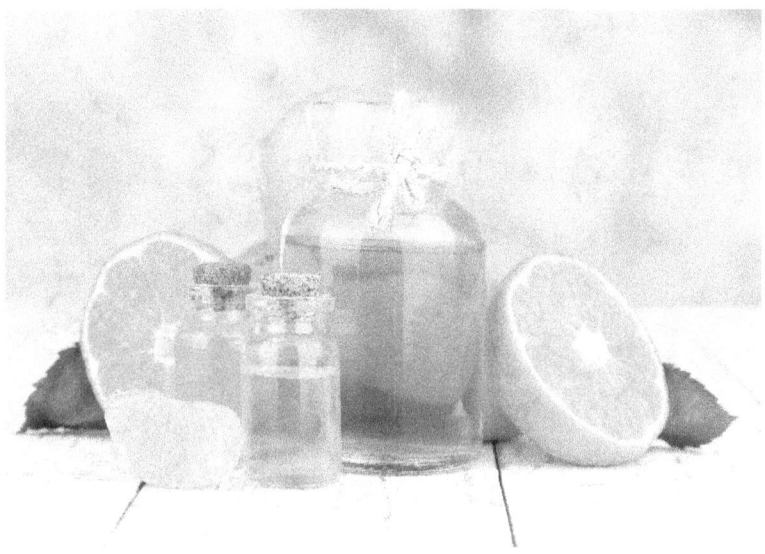

Ingredients:

- 2 tablespoons high-proof vodka
- 20 drops sandalwood essential oil
- 10 drops geranium essential oil
- 5 drops frankincense essential oil
- 5 drops bergamot essential oil

Instructions:

1. Combine the vodka and essential oils in a small spray bottle.
2. Add the water then shake well to combine.
3. Spritz the spray into the air as needed.

Lovely Lavender Bath Salts

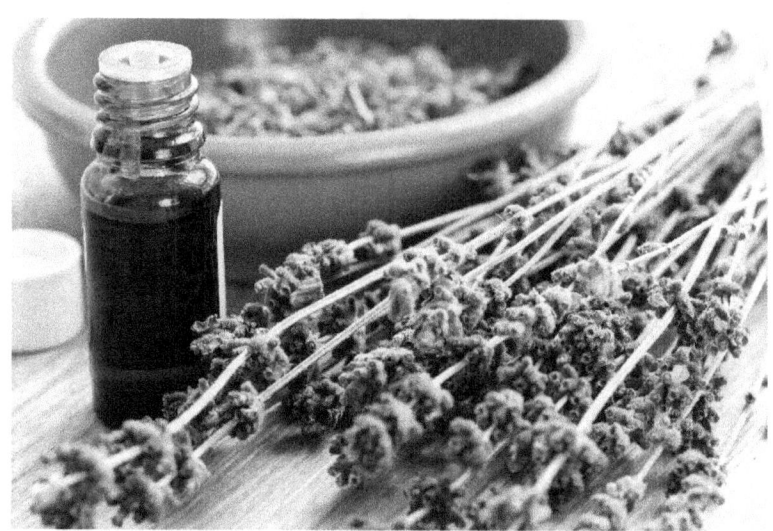

Ingredients:

- 1 ½ cups Epsom salts
- 1 ½ cups coarse Himalayan pink salt
- ½ cup baking soda
- 5 drops lavender essential oil
- 3 drops frankincense essential oil
- 1 drop geranium essential oil

Instructions:

1. Combine the Epsom salts, Himalayan salt and baking soda in a large bowl.
2. Stir until well combined then add the essential oils.
3. Use a metal spoon to stir the ingredients together then store in a dark glass jar.

4. Cover the jar with the lid and let the oils blend for at least 24 hours
5. To use the bath salts, draw a hot bath and stir in 1 cup of bath salt until thoroughly dissolved.
6. Soak for at least 30 minutes then towel dry.

Feeling Free Diffuser Blend

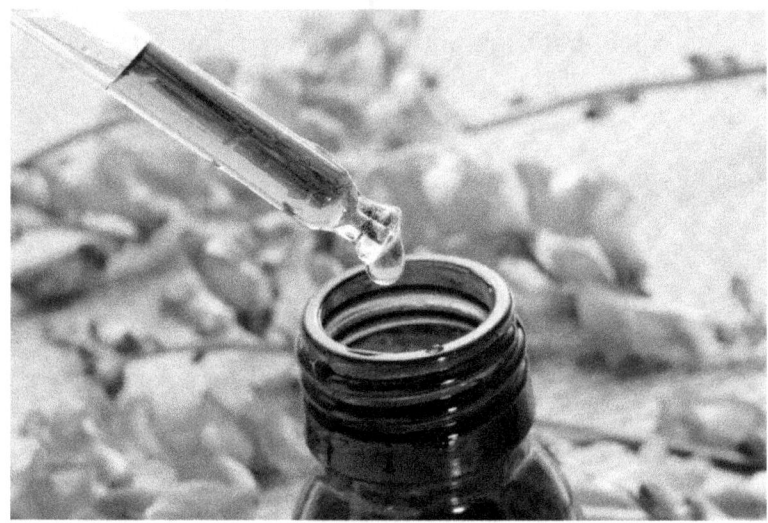

Ingredients:

- ¼ cup sweet almond oil
- 1 tablespoon high-proof vodka
- ½ teaspoon frankincense essential oil
- ¼ teaspoon geranium essential oil
- ¼ teaspoon neroli essential oil

Instructions:

1. Combine the sweet almond oil, vodka, and essential oils in a glass bottle.
2. Place the cap on the bottle and swirl gently to combine the ingredients.
3. Remove the cap and place several diffuser reeds in the bottle.

4. Let the reeds soak until saturated then turn them over to put the dry ends in the bottle.

Frankincense Healing Salve for Burns and Cuts

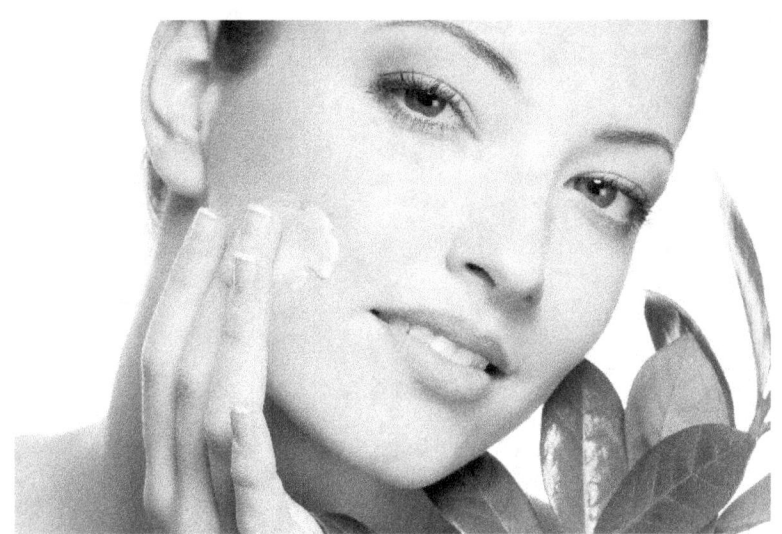

Ingredients:

- ¼ cup extra-virgin olive oil
- ¼ cup cold-pressed coconut oil
- 1 tablespoon beeswax granules
- 4 drops lavender essential oil
- 2 drops lemon essential oil
- 1 drop frankincense essential oil
- 1 drop vitamin E oil

Instructions:

1. Combine the olive oil, coconut oil and beeswax in a double boiler over low heat.

2. Warm the mixture until it is melted then stir well.
3. Combine the essential oils and vitamin E oil in a small glass jar.
4. Pour in the melted mixture and swirl to combine.
5. Let the jar set at room temperature until it solidifies.
6. Use the salve as needed for burns, cuts, and other minor injuries.

Restful Relaxation Bath Oil

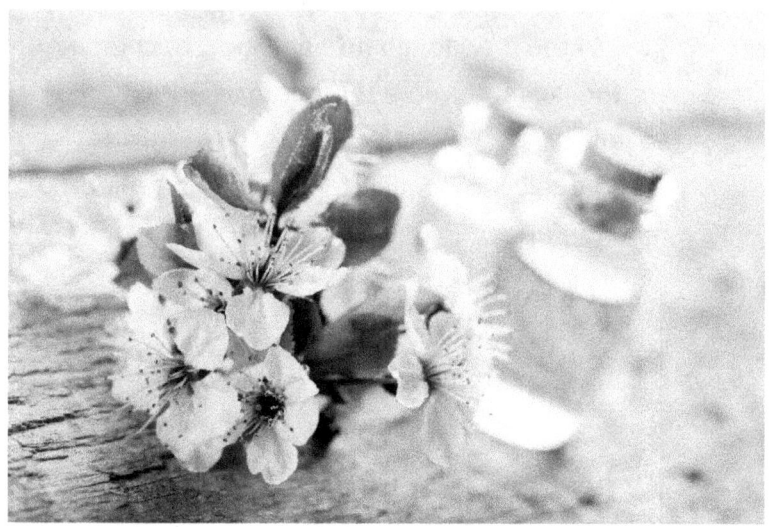

Ingredients:

- 10 drops bergamot essential oil
- 4 drops frankincense essential oil
- 4 drops geranium essential oil
- 2 drops jasmine essential oil
- ½ cup sweet almond oil

Instructions:

1. Combine all of the essential oils in a small dark glass bottle.
2. Swirl the oils gently to combine then add the sweet almond oil and swirl again.
3. To use the oils, run a hot bath then add up to 1 tablespoon of the bath oil.

4. Stir the water gently by hand to disperse the oils.
5. Soak for at least 30 minutes then towel dry.

Mood-Balancing Massage Oil

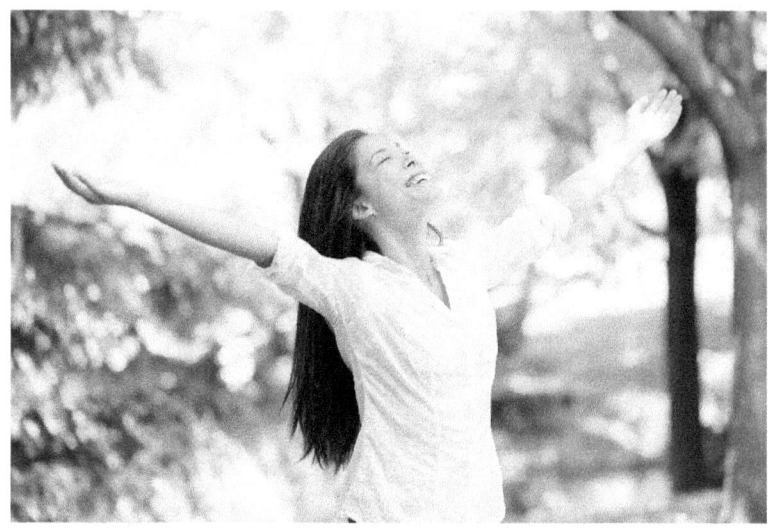

Ingredients:

- ¼ cup jojoba oil
- 4 drops frankincense essential oil
- 3 drops clary sage essential oil
- 3 drops bergamot essential oil

Instructions:

1. Combine the ingredients in a dark glass bottle.
2. Swirl gently to combine the oils then store with the lid on.
3. Let the oils blend for 24 hours then test for fragrance.
4. Apply the massage oil to bare skin and massage it in by hand.

Spiritual Awakening Bath Salts

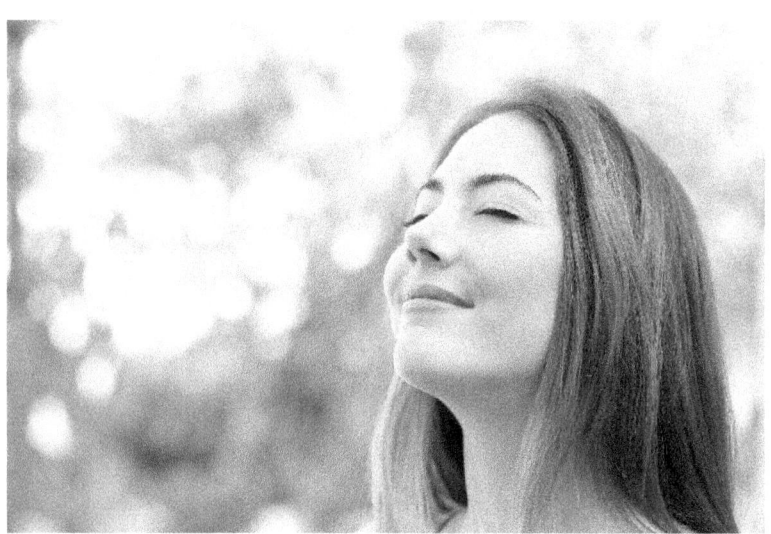

Ingredients:

- 2 cups Epsom salts
- 1 cup coarse sea salt
- ½ cup baking soda
- 4 drops frankincense essential oil
- 3 drops sandalwood essential oil
- 1 drop cedarwood essential oil

Instructions:

1. Combine the Epsom salts, Himalayan salt and baking soda in a large bowl.
2. Stir until well combined then add the essential oils.
3. Use a metal spoon to stir the ingredients together then store in a dark glass jar.

4. Cover the jar with the lid and let the oils blend for at least 24 hours
5. To use the bath salts, draw a hot bath and stir in 1 cup of bath salt until thoroughly dissolved.
6. Soak for at least 30 minutes then towel dry.

Nerve-Calming Inhalation

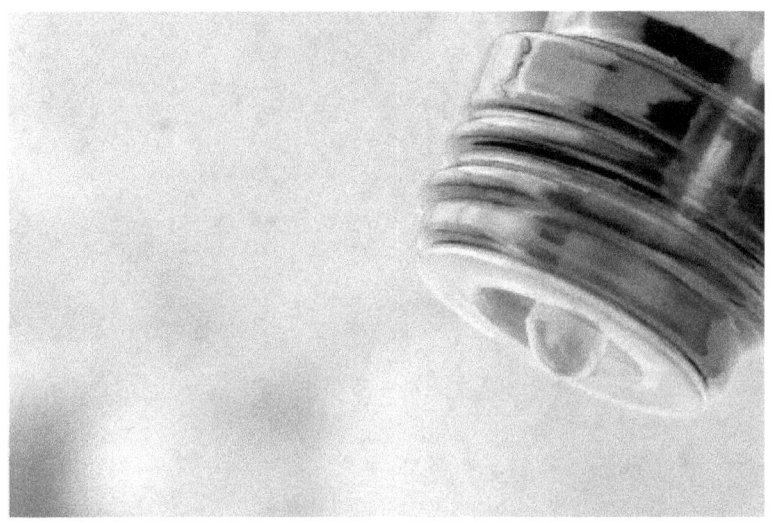

Ingredients:

- 2 to 3 drops frankincense essential oil
- 2 to 3 drops sandalwood essential oil

Instructions:

3. Add the essential oil drops to a clean cloth or tissue.
4. Place the cloth under your nose and inhale deeply.

Sleep-Promoting Room Spray

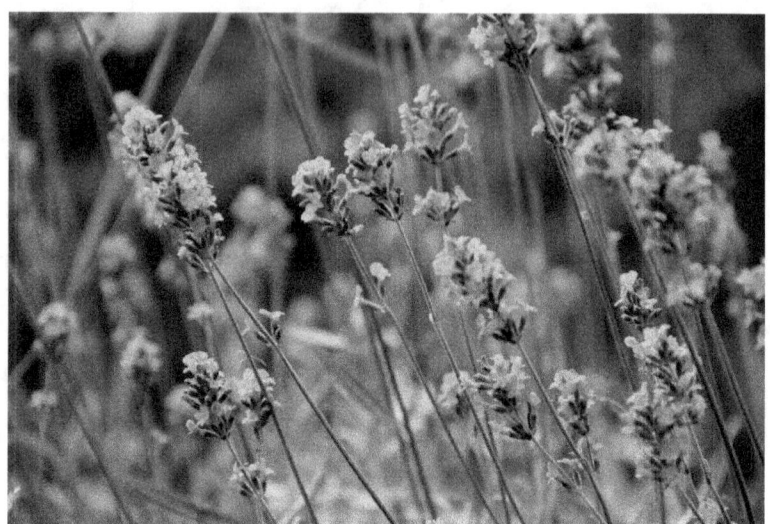

Ingredients:

- 2 tablespoons high-proof vodka
- 20 drops lavender essential oil
- 10 drops sandalwood essential oil
- 5 drops frankincense essential oil
- 5 drops ylang ylang essential oil

Instructions:

1. Combine the vodka and essential oils in a small spray bottle.
2. Add the water then shake well to combine.
3. Spritz the spray into the air as needed.

Frankincense Toothpaste for Oral Pain

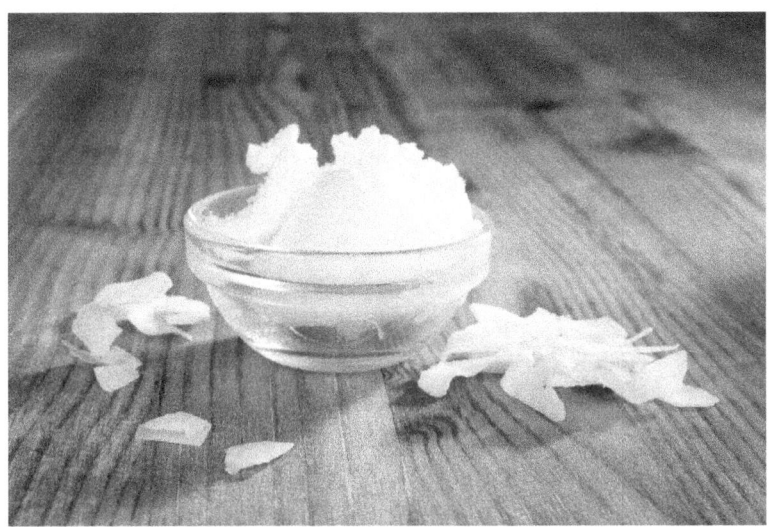

Ingredients:

- 5 teaspoons calcium powder
- 3 teaspoons xylitol powder (or other powdered sweetener)
- 2 teaspoons baking soda
- 1 tablespoon coconut oil
- 2 to 4 drops frankincense essential oil

Instructions:

1. Combine the powdered ingredients in a small bowl and stir well.
2. Stir in the coconut oil until the desired consistency is reached.

3. Add the essential oils then spoon into a glass jar and store with the lid on.
4. To use, apply a small amount to a toothbrush and use as normal.

Moisturizing Floral Facial Cream

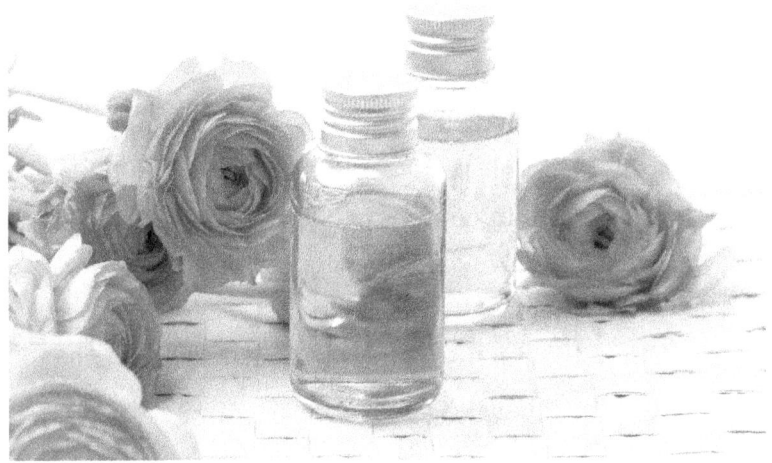

Ingredients:

- 6 tablespoons sweet almond oil
- 2 tablespoons emulsifying wax
- 2 ½ tablespoons vegetable glycerin
- ½ teaspoon stearic acid
- 1 teaspoon vitamin E oil
- 6 tablespoons geranium hydrosol
- 6 tablespoons rose hydrosol, or rose water
- 2 tablespoons aloe vera gel
- 10 drops grapefruit seed extract
- 6 drops rose essential oil
- 4 drops frankincense essential oil
- 4 drops lavender essential oil

- 2 drops geranium essential oil

Instructions:

1. Combine the sweet almond oil, emulsifying wax, vegetable glycerin and stearic acid in a double boiler over low heat.
2. Warm the mixture until the wax melts then remove from heat.
3. Stir in the vitamin E oil then set aside to cool.
4. In a microwave-safe bowl, combine the hydrosols with the aloe vera gel.
5. Warm the mixture until it is lukewarm then stir it into the oil mixture.
6. Add the essential oils and grapefruit seed extract, stirring well.
7. Pour the mixture into an 8-ounce dark glass bottle and cool to room temperature.
8. Put the lid on the jar and store in a cool, dark area – shake before using.

Pain-Relieving Bath Oil Blend

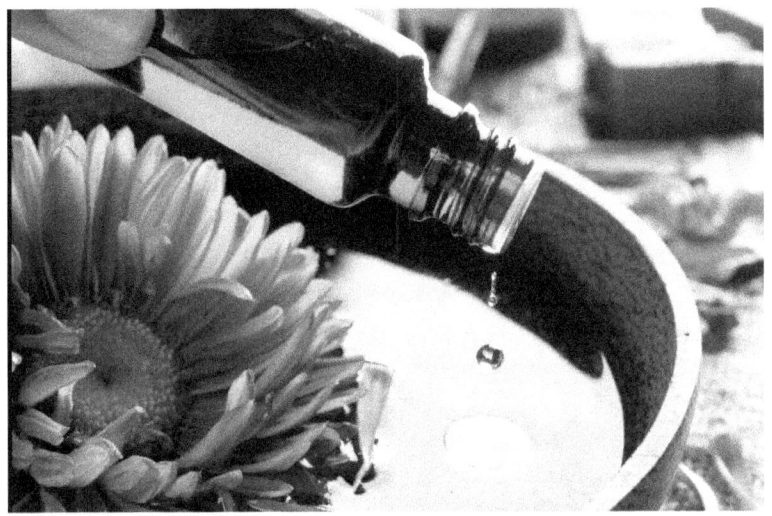

Ingredients:

- 6 drops marjoram essential oil
- 4 drops lavender essential oil
- 4 drops frankincense essential oil
- 2 drops cedarwood essential oil
- ½ cup jojoba oil

Instructions:

1. Combine all of the essential oils in a small dark glass bottle.
2. Swirl the oils gently to combine then add the jojoba oil and swirl again.
3. To use the oils, run a hot bath then add up to 1 tablespoon of the bath oil.

4. Stir the water gently by hand to disperse the oils.
5. Soak for at least 30 minutes then towel dry.

Immune-Boosting Diffuser Blend

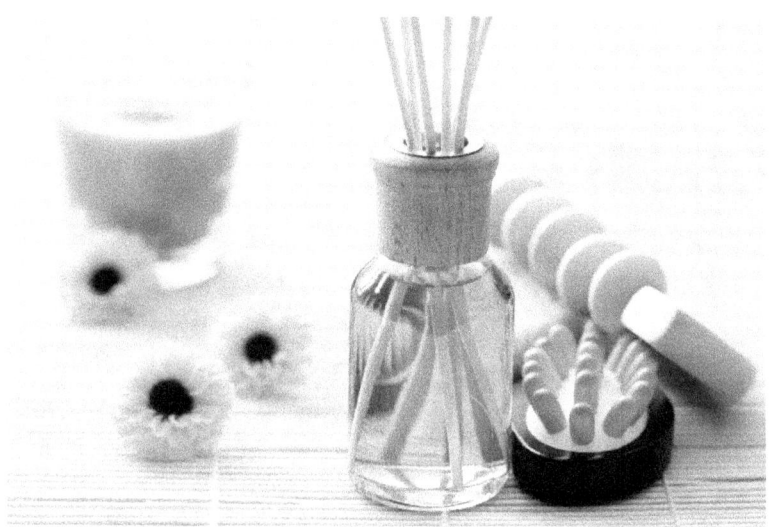

Ingredients:

- ¼ cup sweet almond oil
- 1 tablespoon high-proof vodka
- ½ teaspoon frankincense essential oil
- ¼ teaspoon lemon essential oil
- ¼ teaspoon lavender essential oil

Instructions:

1. Combine the sweet almond oil, vodka, and essential oils in a glass bottle.
2. Place the cap on the bottle and swirl gently to combine the ingredients.
3. Remove the cap and place several diffuser reeds in the bottle.

4. Let the reeds soak until saturated then turn them over to put the dry ends in the bottle.

Conclusion

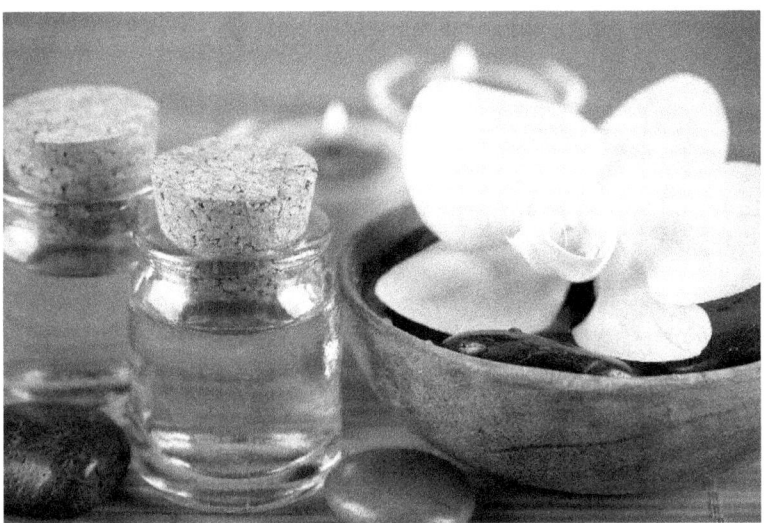

By now, you should have a thorough understanding of what frankincense essential oil is, where it comes from and how it can be used. This wonderful oil has a nice earthy aroma, and it has many health benefits to offer. Not only can you use essential oil in diffuser recipes, but you can put its medicinal benefits to use in homemade salves, oils and balms. If you are ready to try frankincense essential oil for yourself, simply pick a recipe from this book and get going!

www.ingramcontent.com/pod-product-compliance
Lightning Source LLC
Chambersburg PA
CBHW071253280526
45788CB00004B/1704